Most of us have heard of the Black Dog metaphor for Depression. However, mental illness disorders of Anxiety and Depression commonly coexist, so I like to call the Anxiety-Depression combination the Grey-Black Dog; whether it's Anxiety as prominent, leading to depressive or withdrawal episodes, or Depression as primary with bouts of, or together with Anxiety.

Greetings…

I am honoured that you have chosen *Dad's Weird Frown* to help **Approach, Explain** and **Understand** the struggles of mental health. When reading this book, treat it as a guide, replacing or adding other examples relevant to your situation, and interchange the words 'dad/mum' and 'him/her' as required.

I hope these ideas offer understanding and knowledge, to help make a positive impact within relationships. The emotional pain of mental illness, affects more than just the sufferer. The hurt spreads outward like ripples in water, touching the lives of others who are close.

If a heart is locked up with past hurts, may these fresh insights encourage candid conversations, to help break down the barriers, and provide a way forward towards the unlocking power of forgiveness.

While reading or listening, be open-minded as you journey through your thoughts and feelings, with the possibility of similar struggles, not only in your own life, but that of your spouse, loved ones or friends.

Special Thanks To …
My two beautiful, insightful daughters Bethany and Esther, for helping me with the creation of *Dad's Weird Frown*.

Ruth

Copyright ©2024 Ruth Parfett

All rights reserved. No part of this book may be used or reproduced by any means, graphic, electronic, or mechanical, including photocopying, recording, taping or by any information storage retrieval system without the written permission of the author, except in the case of brief cited quotations embodied in articles or reviews.

The content in this book does not constitute medical advice and should not be relied on as such. All content and media are published for informational and educational purposes only and is not tailored to the personal circumstances of any individual. You should always consult a medical professional or healthcare provider if you are seeking medical advice, diagnoses, or treatment.

All illustrations herein, were created and provided by Ruth Parfett. Any persons depicted are being used solely for illustrative purposes only and are not a direct representation of any individual.

Pebble Collections, Print Information: Print ISBN 978-0-6484553-2-5
Ebook ISBN 978-0-6484553-3-2

Because of the dynamic nature of the Internet, any web addresses or links contained in this book may have changed since publication and may no longer be valid.

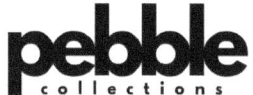

www.pebblecollections.com

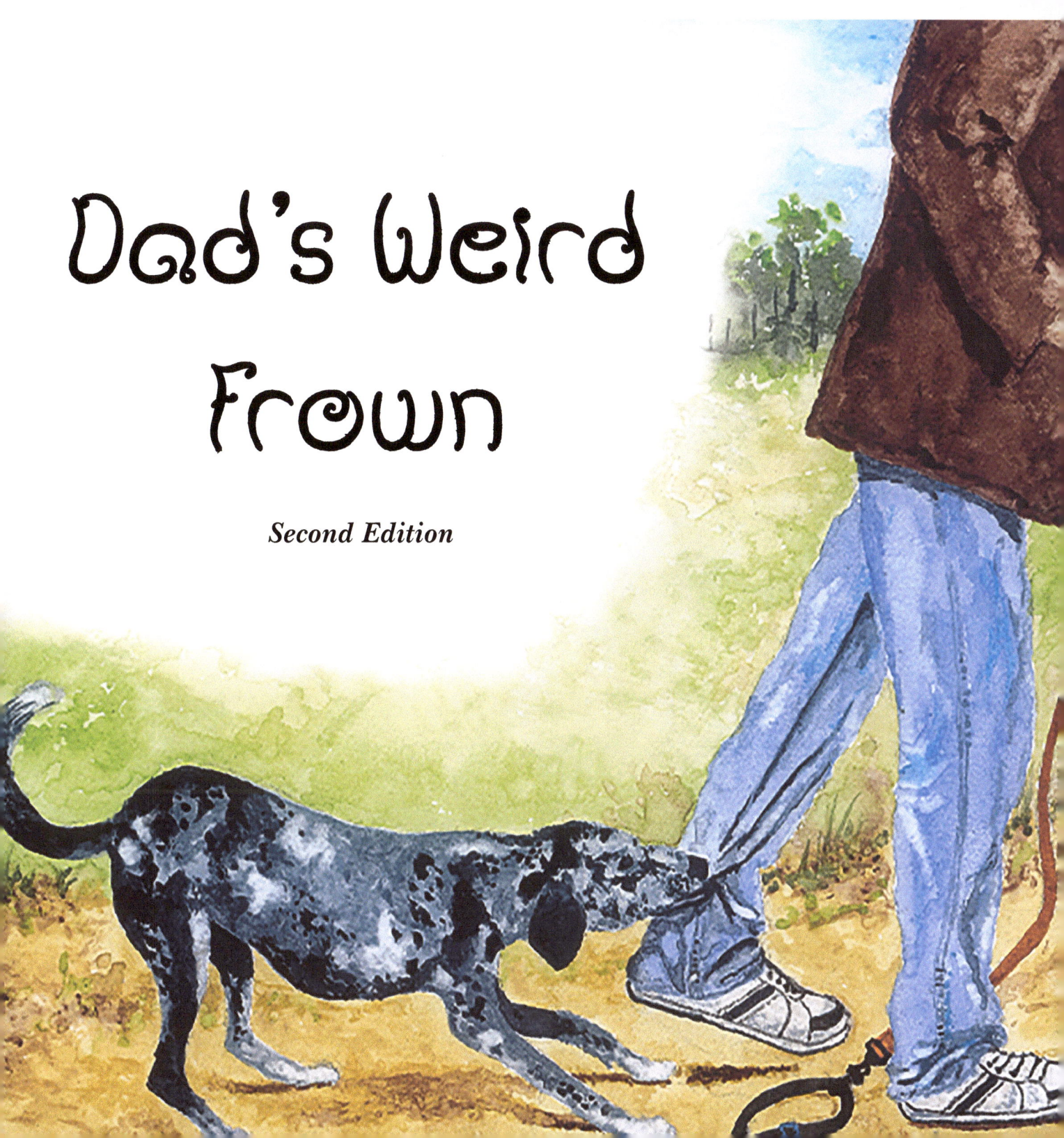

Hi, my name is Ruth.

I would like to write to you about some strange *behaviours* with your dad. These behaviours you might have noticed and some I explain, may not be right for him. Have a little think with your mum, about some of the examples I give in this book, as I share with you.

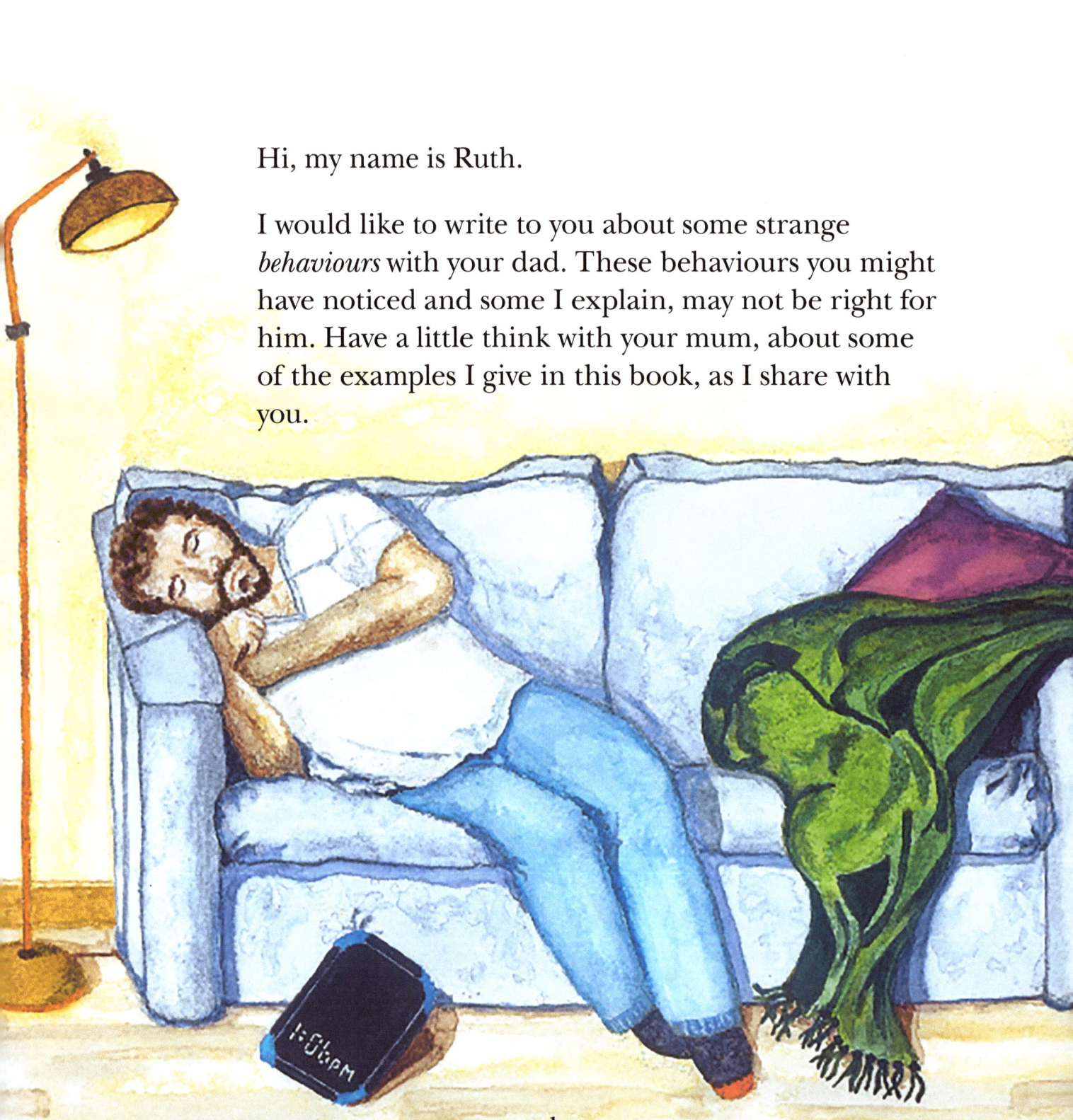

Does it seem your dad is grumpy-dumpy more often than he is happy? Perhaps you feel like you need to check with mum if he *is* happy, before you ask him to do something for you?

Maybe he seems sad a lot. Like his happy-self has gone away on lots of short, sometimes long holidays without you?

Does he seem always tired or sleep during strange times of the day that are not normal bedtimes? He might sleep on his bed or in his usual chair.

Possibly he has stopped working in his favourite workspace, leaving jobs he would normally finish left not done.

Or maybe he does not like going to places he used to enjoy? Can you think of some?

How about going out at night to dinner with the family?

He may no longer enjoy spending time with his friends.

Or he does not like people visiting your home anymore?

Instead, he may prefer to be alone, watch television, movies or play computer games all the time.

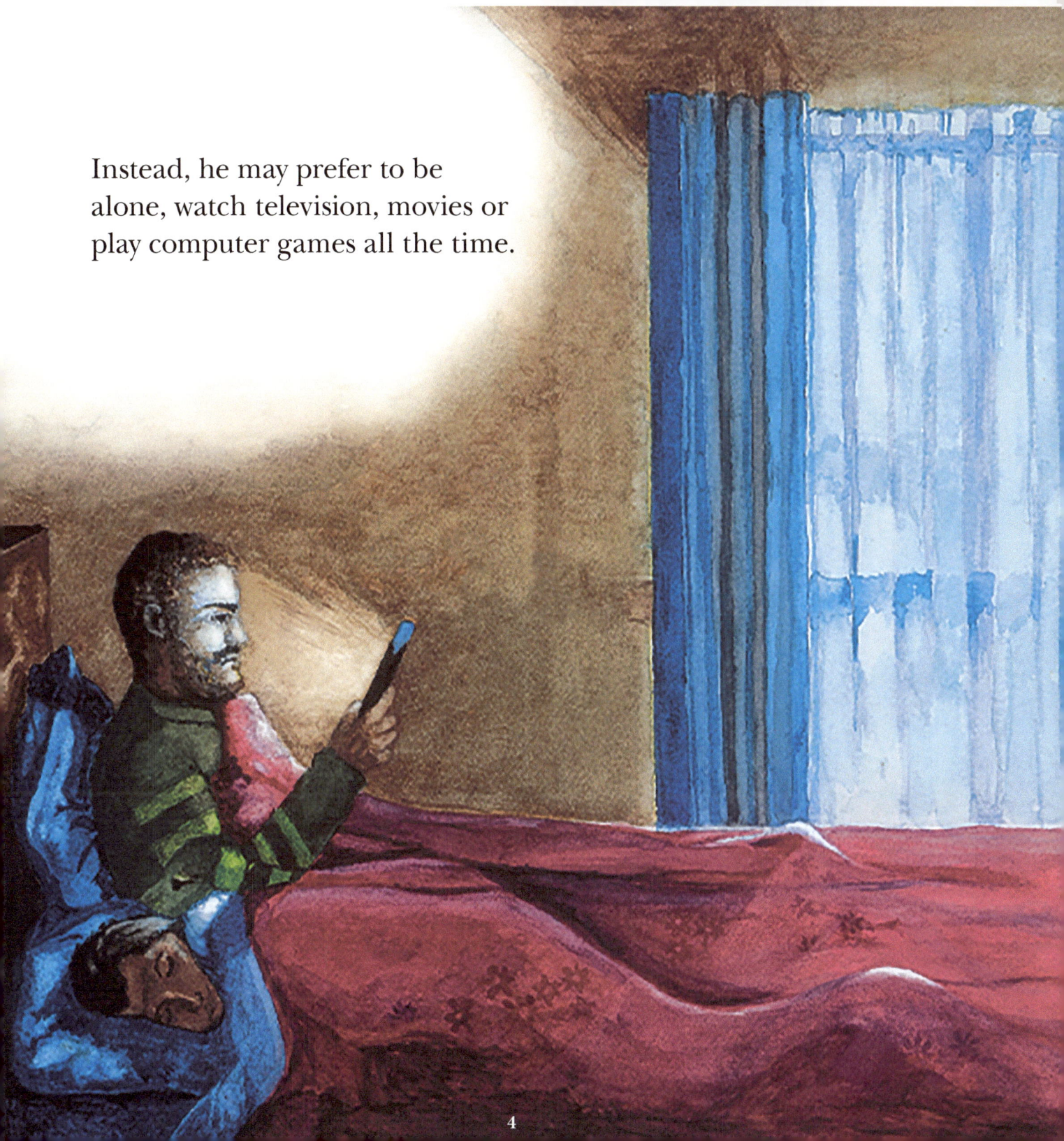

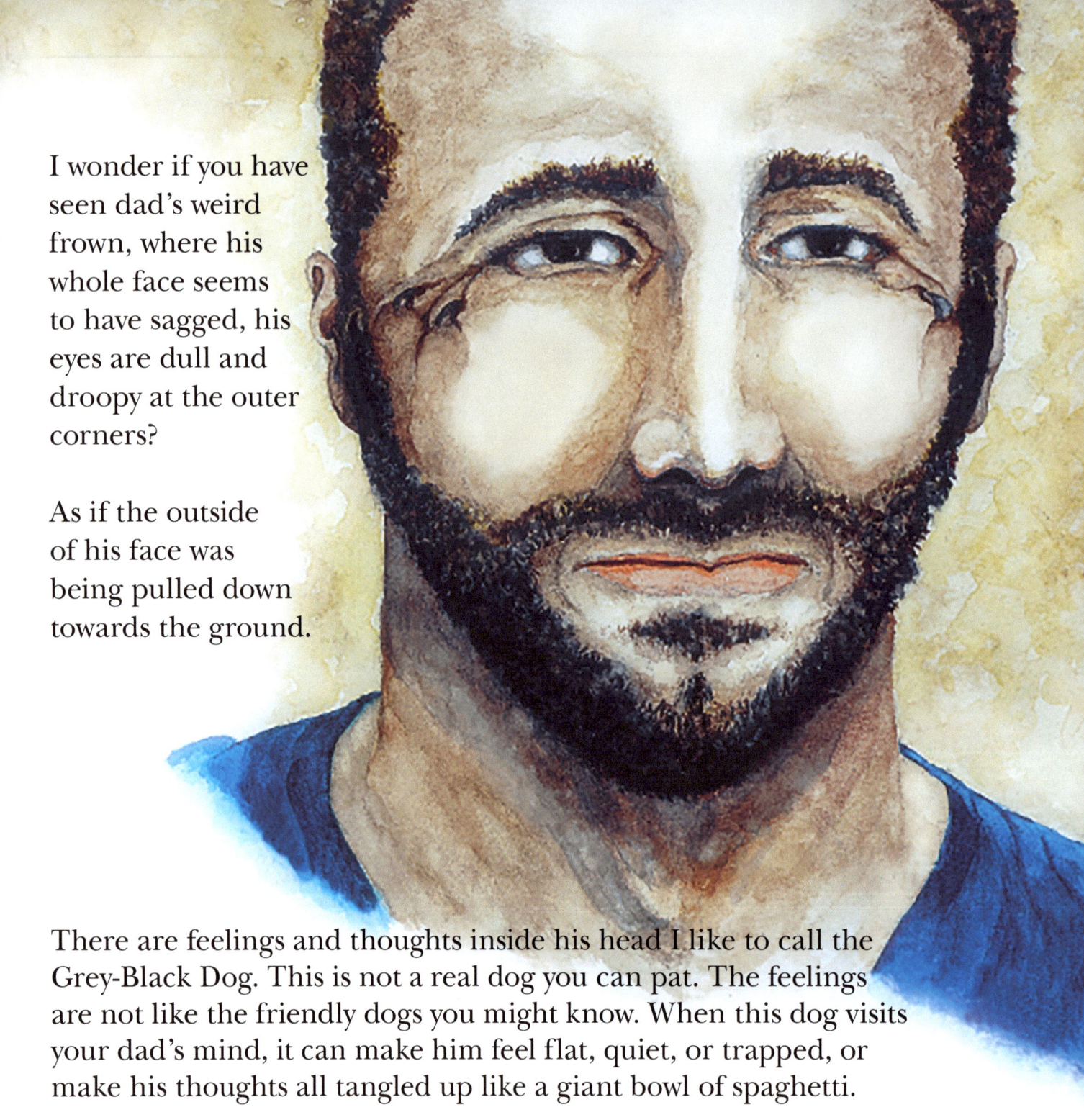

I wonder if you have seen dad's weird frown, where his whole face seems to have sagged, his eyes are dull and droopy at the outer corners?

As if the outside of his face was being pulled down towards the ground.

There are feelings and thoughts inside his head I like to call the Grey-Black Dog. This is not a real dog you can pat. The feelings are not like the friendly dogs you might know. When this dog visits your dad's mind, it can make him feel flat, quiet, or trapped, or make his thoughts all tangled up like a giant bowl of spaghetti.

This dog can hide in all areas of your dad's life, like the dogs I've hidden within some of these pictures I've painted.

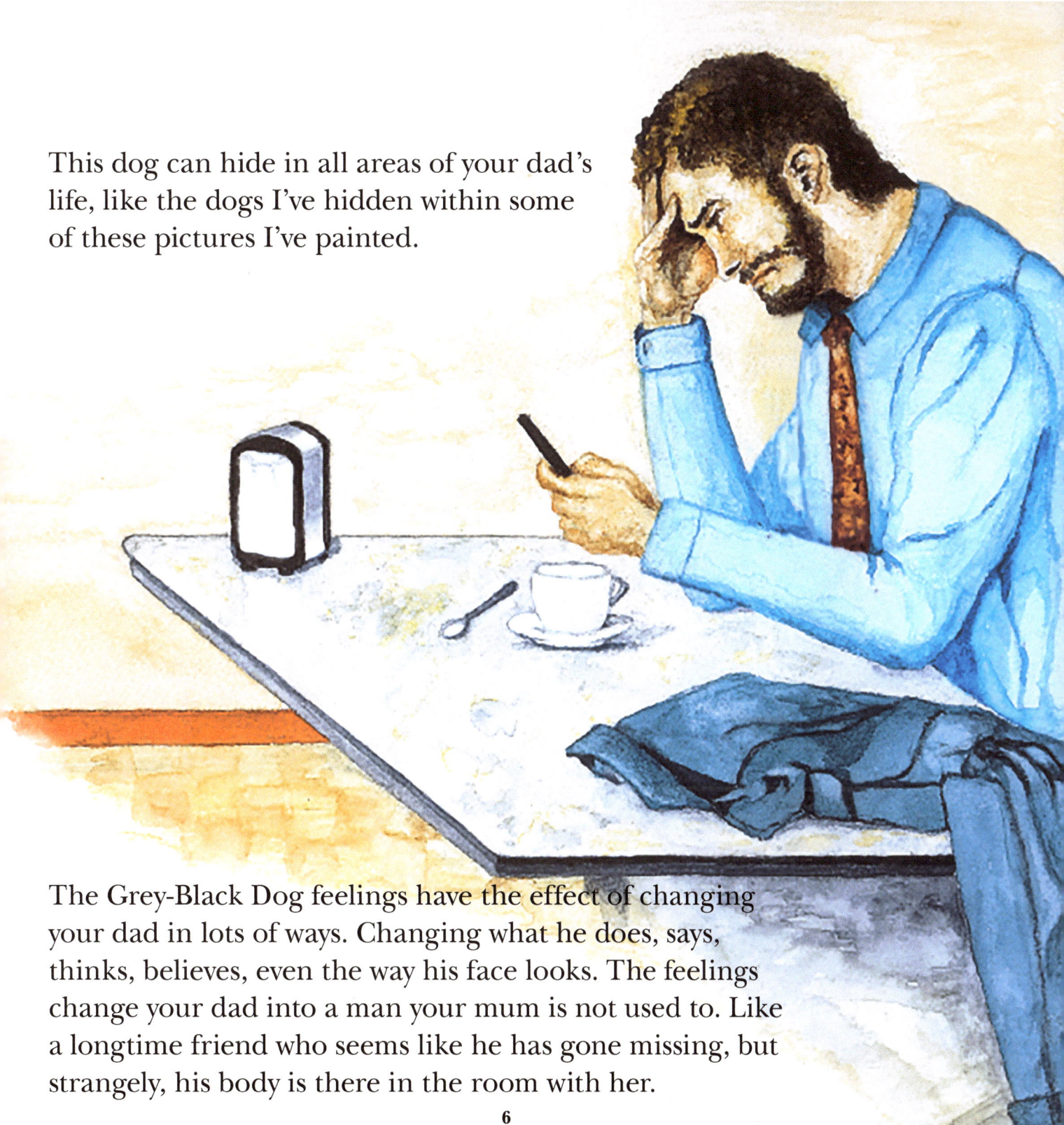

The Grey-Black Dog feelings have the effect of changing your dad in lots of ways. Changing what he does, says, thinks, believes, even the way his face looks. The feelings change your dad into a man your mum is not used to. Like a longtime friend who seems like he has gone missing, but strangely, his body is there in the room with her.

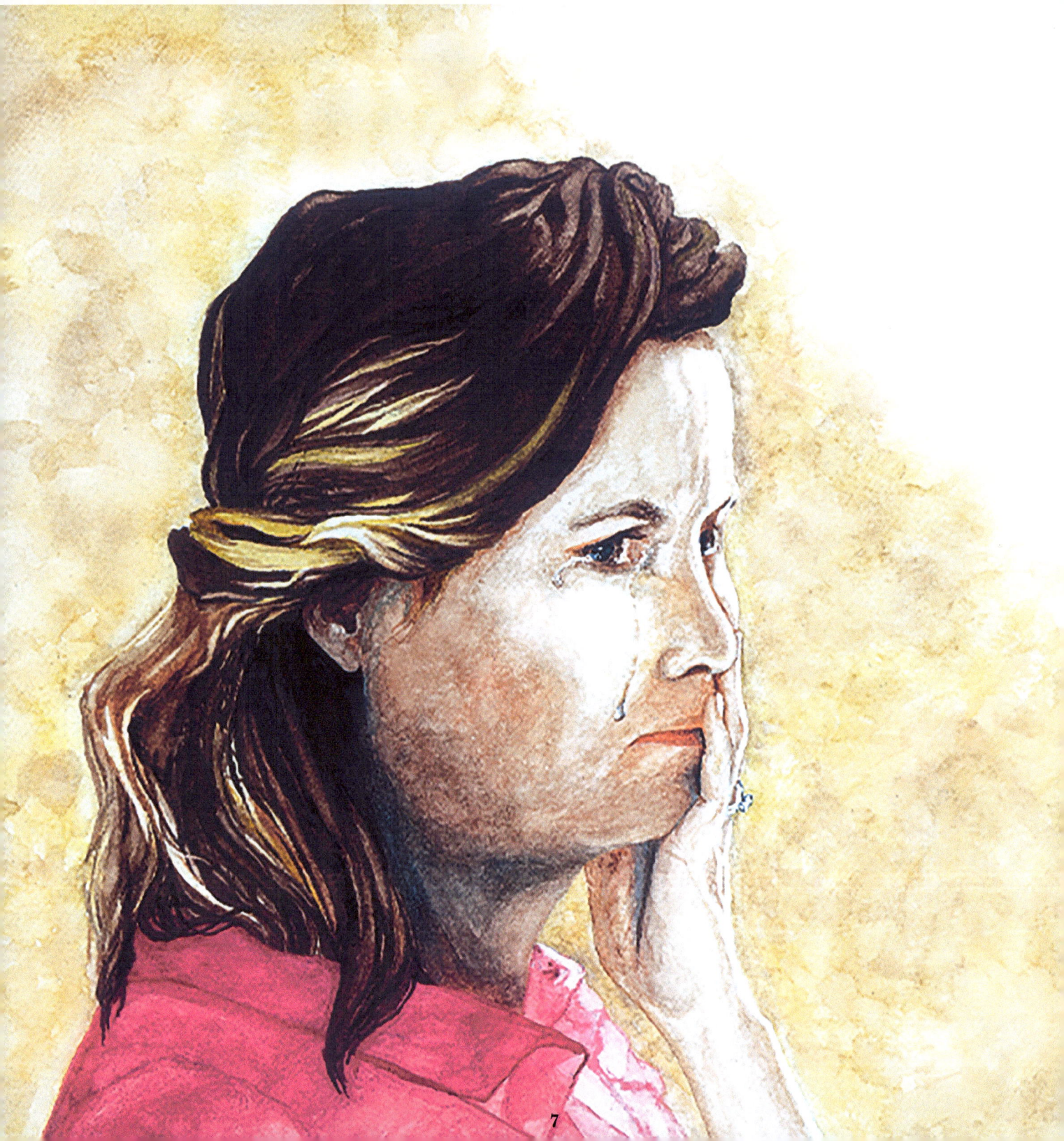

Have you seen your dad get grumpy at your mum and make her cry? Let me whisper you a little secret. It is not because of you.

Your mum is sad because she misses your dad, her best friend, *so* much. She misses the way he used to be before the feelings changed him.

You need to know that when your dad is being any or all those strange behaviours I have talked about, it means he is struggling with those feelings in his head. Making him irritable, and act in a way he might not be aware of, from feelings he may not fully understand.

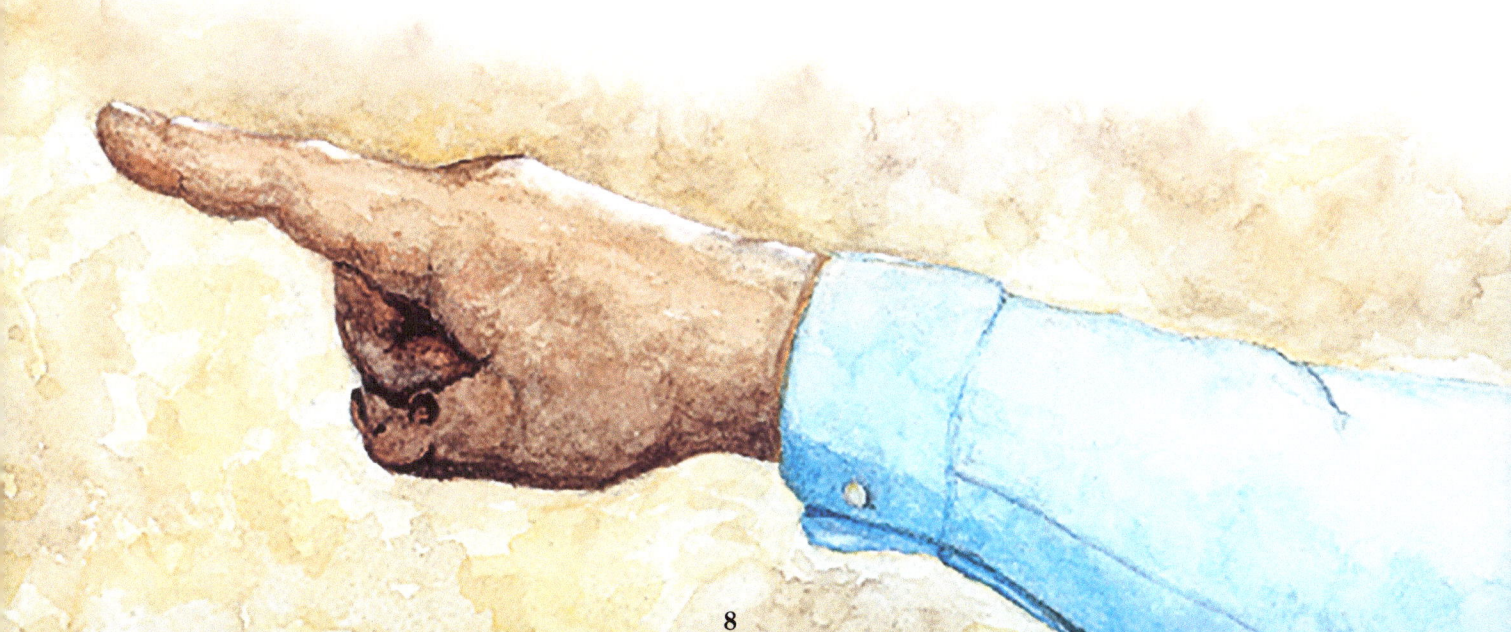

When he struggles, his mind is like driving through thick fog. Everything slows down because he cannot see too far ahead. When we try to see through fog, everything is smudged and blurry, making it hard to spot obstacles like other cars, animals, or road signs.

When dad has these fog-like feelings inside his head, it can be hard for him to see and feel his thoughts clearly. This makes it hard for him to know which way to go or the right choices to make.

Living life through large patches of this mind fog, is very tiring and frustrating for him. It seems as if all his strength to do things, is draining out of him and leaving his energy tank empty. This might be why your dad sleeps a lot. Maybe why he gets grumpy at you or your mum. Or it might be why your dad does not like visiting friends or family like you remember he used to.

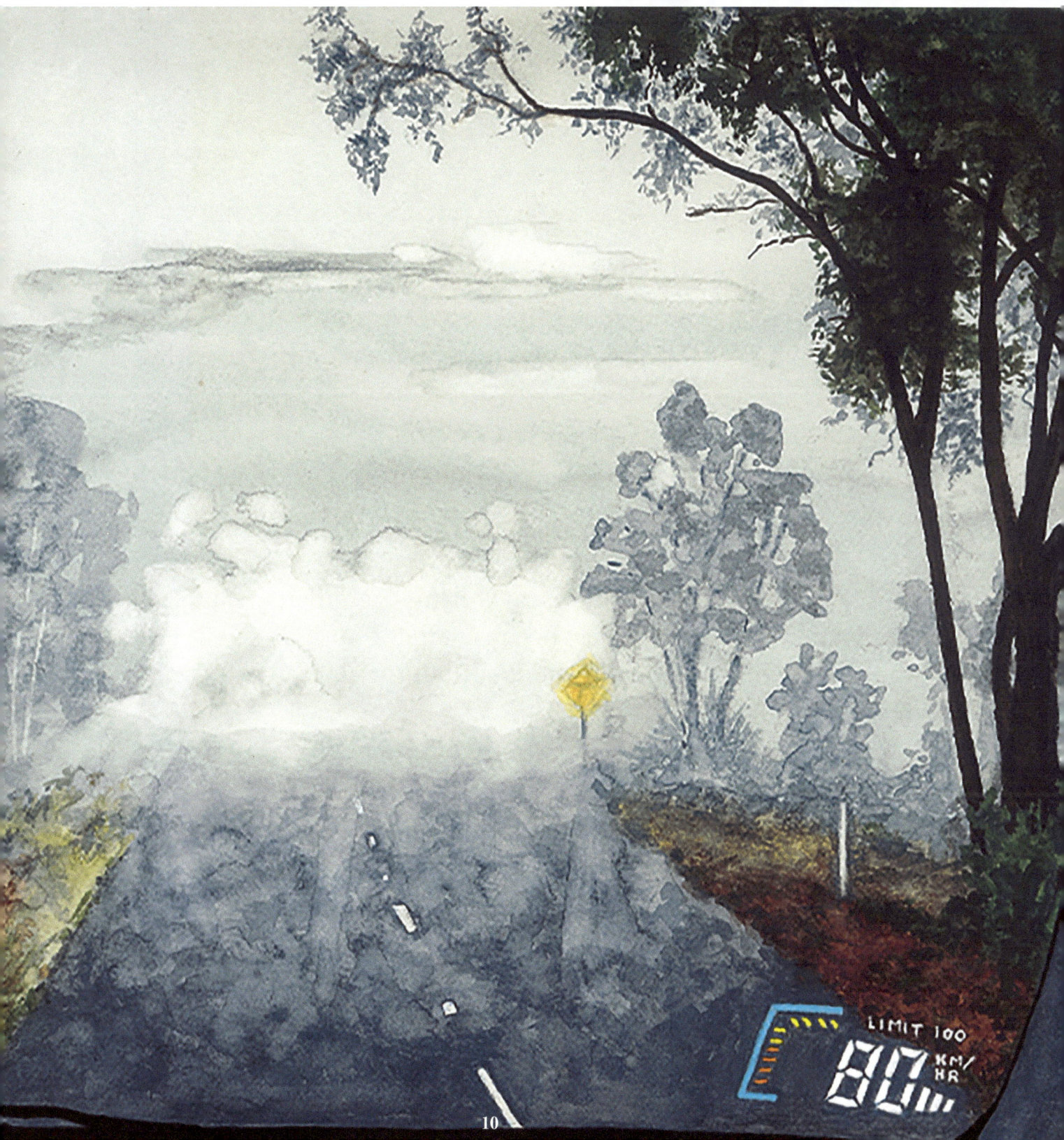

You and your mum might see all these behaviours in your dad. But he might not. So, I need you to listen to me very carefully.

If you are confused, have questions that bother you or feelings you do not understand, please talk to someone who can help explain them to you. Do not try and work it out all on your own.

If it feels like your dad is far away during these behaviours and not listening to you, it is not because he does not love you. His love for you is deep down inside, past all the doggy, fog-like feelings in his head.

It may be that he feels so weighed down by his struggles, that he finds it very hard to show the love he has for you, in a way that you would recognise.

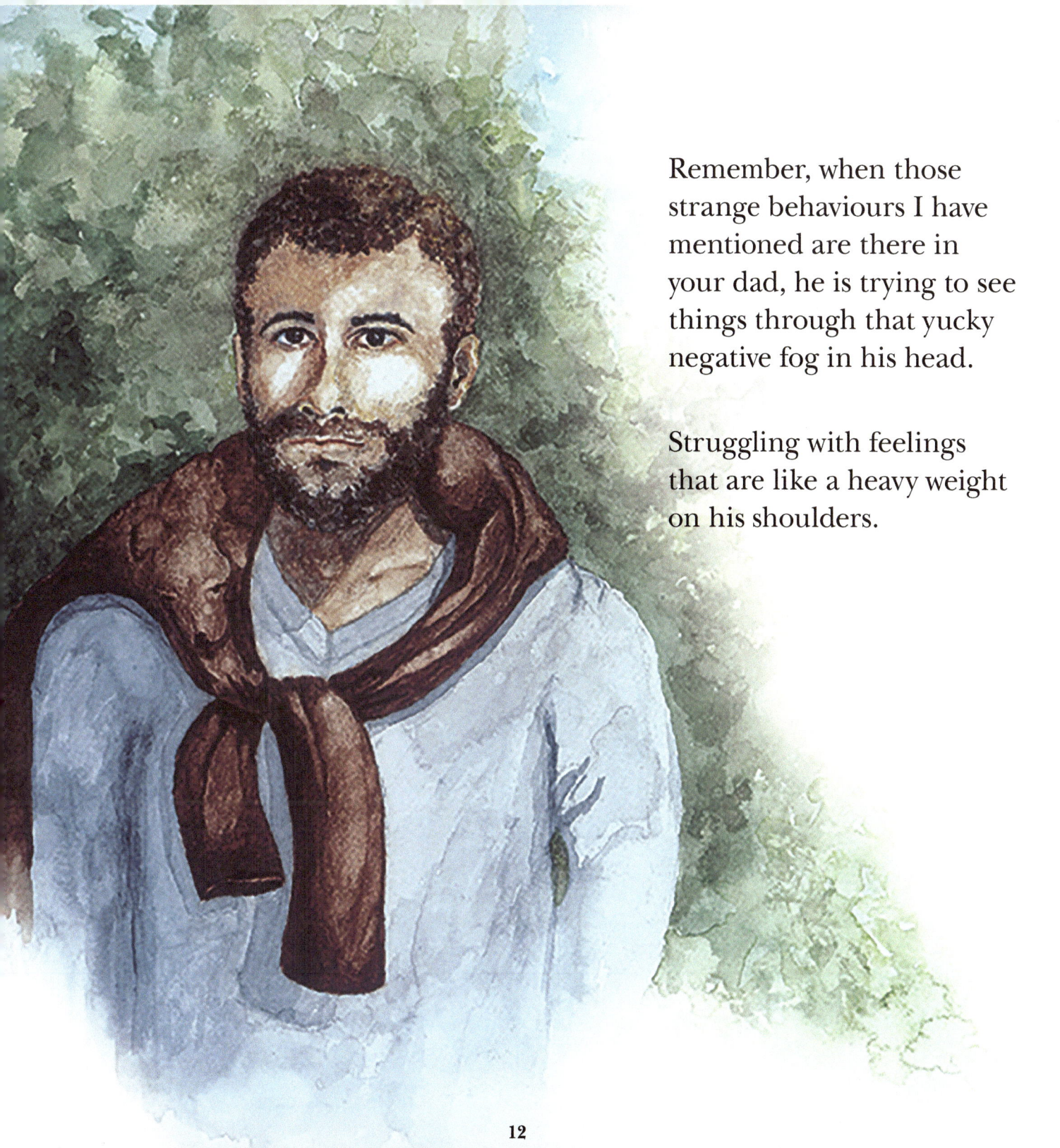

Remember, when those strange behaviours I have mentioned are there in your dad, he is trying to see things through that yucky negative fog in his head.

Struggling with feelings that are like a heavy weight on his shoulders.

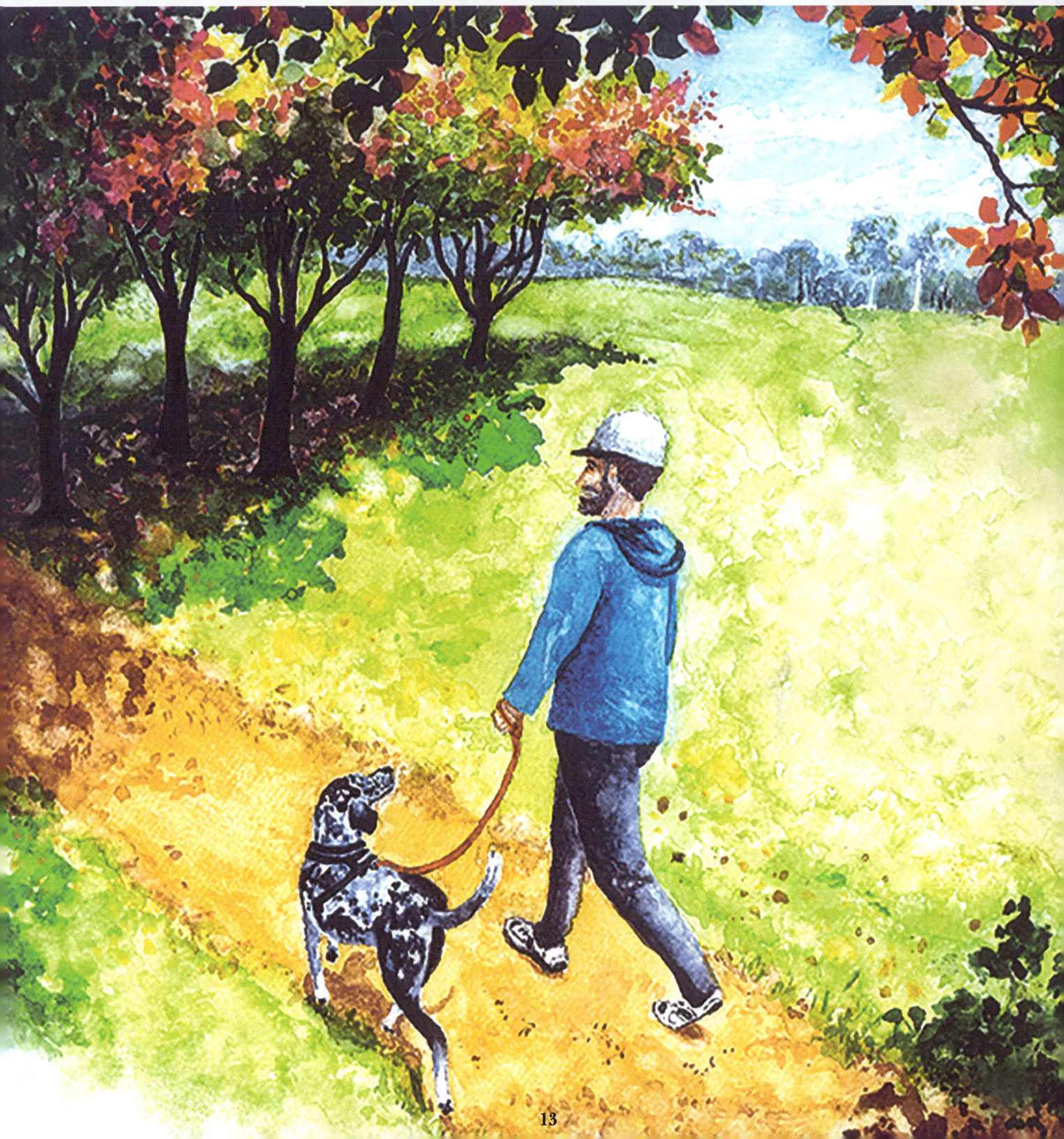

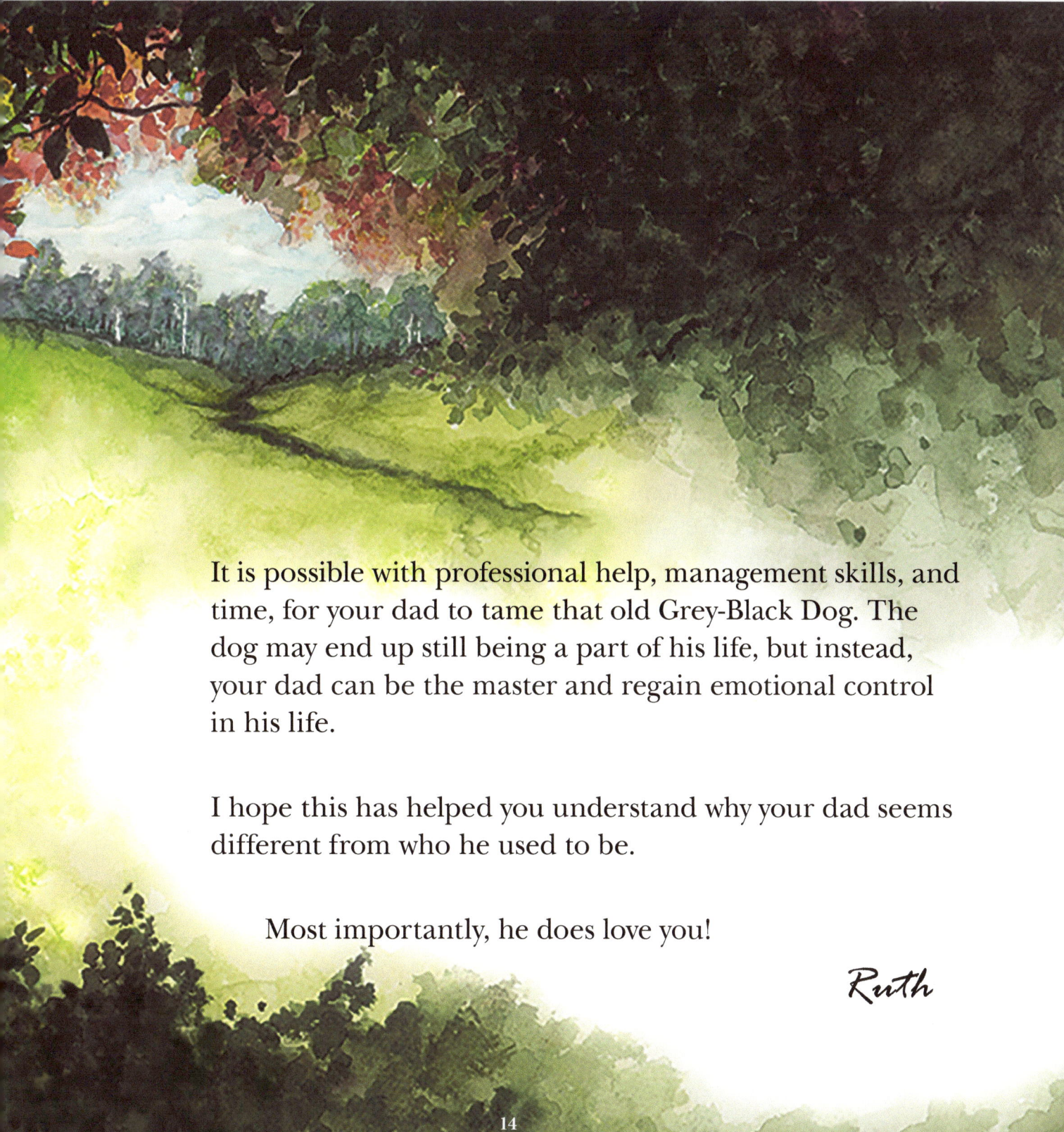

It is possible with professional help, management skills, and time, for your dad to tame that old Grey-Black Dog. The dog may end up still being a part of his life, but instead, your dad can be the master and regain emotional control in his life.

I hope this has helped you understand why your dad seems different from who he used to be.

Most importantly, he does love you!

Ruth

Pebble Collections is designed to help *Unlock Hearts with Pebbles of Hope*. Each of my pebbles are created to reach out with a special message to inspire positivity, courage, contemplation, learning and understanding.

Dad's Weird Frown is one of these Pebbles. Created to help those touched by mental illness and domestic violence, to better approach, explain and understand these complex subjects, in a non-confrontational way.

Visit www.pebblecollections.com to discover more *Pebbles* on offer.

Print Information

Print ISBN 978-0-6484553-2-5
Ebook ISBN 978-0-6484553-3-2

www.ingramcontent.com/pod-product-compliance
Lightning Source LLC
Chambersburg PA
CBHW041203040526
44107CB00090BA/1556